OSTEOPOROSIS DIET

Your Complete Guide to Prevent and Reverse Bone Loss using Natural Remedies, Diet and Exercise without Medication

Includes Healthy Bone Recipes!

Copyright © 2016 Kasia Roberts, RN
All right reserved.

Disclaimer

The information in this book is not to be used as medical advice. The recipes should be used in combination with guidance from your physician. Please consult your physician before beginning any diet. It is especially important for those with diabetes, and those on medications to consult with their physician before making changes to their diet.

All rights reserved. No part of this publication or the information in it may be quoted from or reproduced in any form by means such as printing, scanning, photocopying or otherwise without prior written permission of the copyright holder.

Disclaimer and Terms of Use: Effort has been made to ensure that the information in this book is accurate and complete, however, the author and the publisher do not warrant the accuracy of the information, text and graphics contained within the book due to the rapidly changing nature of science, research, known and unknown facts and internet. The Author and the publisher do not hold any responsibility for errors, omissions or contrary interpretation of the subject matter herein. This book is presented solely for motivational and informational purposes only.

Table of Contents

Introduction: What is Osteoporosis 4

The Causes and Signs of Osteoporosis 10

The Traditional Methods of Treating Osteoporosis 23

Natural Approaches to Osteoporosis Care 31

Stress Reduction 32

Essential Oils 40

Herbs 43

Quitting Bad Health Habits 46

Your Diet and Osteoporosis: The Nutrition You Need to Build and Repair Bone Health 48
    Easy Bone Building Recipes 59
    Decadent Chocolate Smoothie 60
    Blackberry Papaya Smoothie 62
    Spinach Artichoke Portabellas 64
    Ultimate Stuffed Cheese Quesadilla 67
    Bone Building Salad 70
    Spicy Philly Enchiladas 73
    Stuffed Endive 76
    Spaghetti Squash Italiano 78

Supplements for Osteoporosis Care 81

Keeping Physically Active to Keep Bones Strong 87

Conclusion 95

INTRODUCTION:
What is Osteoporosis

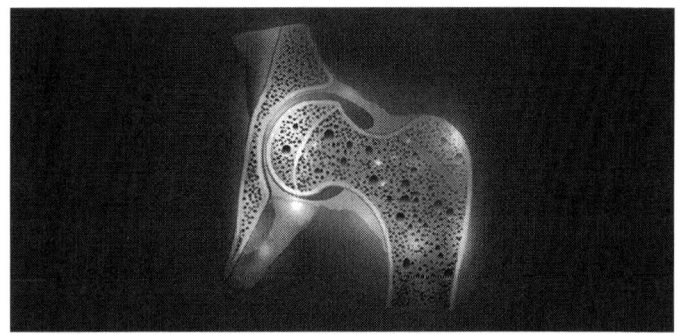

Osteoporosis is a disease that we typically don't give much thought to until we, or someone that we care about, is affected. This is likely because osteoporosis is a disease that generally doesn't strike until middle age begins to set in. By the time that you might start thinking about osteoporosis and the prevention of it, you could already be suffering from the affects of the disease, unknowingly. Knowledge is the number one tool you can have in your arsenal against osteoporosis. When you have the knowledge about what osteoporosis is, how to prevent it and all of the treatment options available to you, both traditional and natural, you can begin to protect your long term bone health and strength.

Osteoporosis is a disease of the skeletal system. During your lifetime, you are constantly losing and rebuilding bone mass. In the earlier decades of life, you build bone mass faster than you lose it, and as a result your bones become thicker and stronger. Most people reach their peak of bone strength and density in their early twenties. As you age, the rate at which you lose bone can match or exceed the rate that you are rebuilding it. This process can become exaggerated due to a variety of factors including genetics, diet and lifestyle. When this happens, the bones become extremely weak and the condition that we call osteoporosis appears.

If you were to take a sample of healthy bone tissue and look at it under a microscope, it would appear somewhat porous, much like a honeycomb. In cases of osteoporosis, when you begin to lose bone mass, the holes in the bone tissue become much larger. This causes the bones to become extremely weak and frail, making you vulnerable to fractures and breaks from even the mildest of stresses.

Osteoporosis is very common. In fact, many people believe that it is an inevitable disease of aging. It is estimated that nearly 55 million Americans over the age of fifty suffer from some degree of osteoporosis. One might think that the fact that it affects so many people would cause us to become more aware, however the opposite seems to have happened. Instead many people take their bone health for granted in their younger years, and take no measures to preserve their strong bones for the future. Often times when an older person begins to complain of back pain, suffers a minor fracture or even seems a little shorter; we simply attribute it to the negative effects of aging.

It is estimated that half of women and twenty-five percent of men over the age of fifty have suffered some type of bone injury due to osteoporosis. The most common types of breaks and fractures from osteoporosis occur in the hips, spine and wrists. This causes not only pain and long recovery times but a diminished quality of life as well. Add to this that nearly one fifth of the people that suffer a broken hip due to the effects of osteoporosis suffer some form of fatal side effect from either the broken bone itself or the surgery that was prescribed to treat it, and osteoporosis suddenly seems much more serious than just some common ailment of aging, as it is often viewed.

The truth is that osteoporosis is preventable and treatable. You do not have to sit back and give in to the effects of osteoporosis. There are a number of ways that you can take back control of your bone health and become stronger than before. It takes a physician to officially diagnose osteoporosis, and you should seek out bone density tests starting as early as your fifties, or even your forties. These tests and assessing your risk for developing osteoporosis is the first step of prevention. The treatments for osteoporosis include traditional medical options, natural alternatives and dietary and lifestyle adaptations. The purpose of this book is to inform you about all of them and also show you how easy it is to build bone mass and prevent future loss by adopting easy lifestyle habits including the best nutrition for bone health.

Osteoporosis is serious and it could cost you with both money and quality of life. There is no reason for you, or someone that you care about, to just sit back and let osteoporosis happen when natural remedies are completely within your reach and easy to adjust to. Here is your opportunity to learn more about osteoporosis and the ways that you can once again stand tall and strong.

The Causes and Signs of Osteoporosis

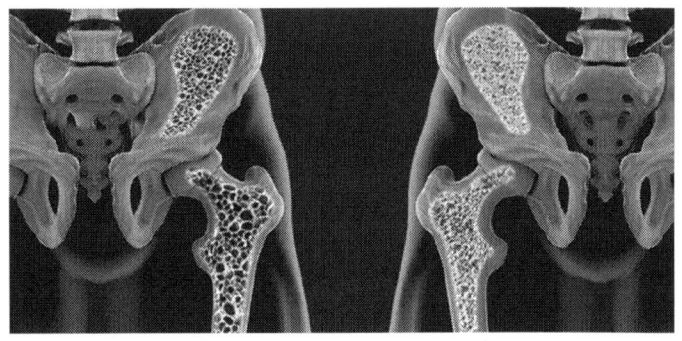

Perhaps one of the most dangerous things about osteoporosis is that it just sneaks up on you. You might be completely unaware that you are suffering from bone loss until the moment your first injury occurs. People with osteoporosis can suffer breaks and fractures from seemingly benign occurrences such as bumping into furniture, a minor fall or even a hard sneeze. The best time to treat osteoporosis is before it begins or before it becomes too severe. Because early treatment is the best treatment, it is important to recognize your risk factors and the early signs of osteoporosis. Here in this section, we will talk about the many factors that can contribute to the onset of osteoporosis and how to recognize the early signs of the disease.

Causes

What causes osteoporosis? There is no simple answer to that question. There is an incredible range of possible contributing factors and it could be any one of them or a combination of them that leads to the development of osteoporosis. The first, and probably the most important, risk factor for osteoporosis is age. Although you reach your peak bone mass in your twenties, it usually isn't until the fifth decade of life that the loss of bone mass becomes a serious issue. It doesn't matter what decade of your life that you are in, taking the measures to prevent your bone health is one of the most important things that you can do. There are also several other leading contributing factors to osteoporosis, including the following.

Gender: Females suffer from bone loss at a rate that more than doubles their male peers. This does not mean that men do not ever suffer from osteoporosis, in fact approximately twenty percent of men aged fifty or older will suffer from osteoporosis to some degree. However, it is estimated that one out of every two women will suffer from osteoporosis. This is likely due to the change in hormone balances that occur with women once they reach menopause.

Race: All races are susceptible to suffering from osteoporosis, however the disease is significantly more common in men and women who are Caucasian or of Asian decent.

Family Health History: There seems to be a greater incidence of osteoporosis occurring among a family tree rather than just random occurrences. If you have a parent or sibling that has osteoporosis you are more likely to suffer from it yourself. This seems to be especially true if the person in your family had osteoporosis that was severe enough to result in a serious injury such as a hip fracture.

Skeletal Size: Both men and women who have smaller skeletal frames are more likely to suffer from osteoporosis than their taller counterparts. The reason for this is actually quite simple. The larger you are, the more bone mass you have. The more bone mass you have, the more you can afford to lose without suffering serious consequences.

Sedentary Living: People who have not made physical fitness a priority or those who have held jobs that required long hours sitting at a desk seem to be at a greater risk of developing osteoporosis. It is known that regular exercise, especially gentle weight bearing exercises can help build bone strength. If you do not regularly commit to these types of exercises, you are more likely to suffer from weakened bone structure.

Bad Lifestyle Habits: Although the connections are not completely understood, it is shown that consuming more than two alcoholic beverages per day and tobacco usage both contribute to the loss of bone mass. The additional inflammation that is caused by these lifestyle habits is suspected to be behind the increased risk.

Lack of Dietary Calcium: Calcium intake is absolutely vital in the building of bone mass during the growth years of childhood and early adulthood. It is equally important for stalling the amount of bone loss that occurs as we age. Adequate calcium intake throughout your entire life is important because you can actually accumulate a bone "bank". By this I mean that if you make bone health a priority early on, your bones will be stronger than someone who didn't make the same choices. This means that you might still lose a normal amount of bone mass as you age, but you had more mass to begin with so the effects of the loss will be less noticeable.

Vitamin D Deficiency: Vitamin D is important for the absorption and utilization of calcium. Without it, it is impossible for your body to make the most of the calcium it does take in. Because so many people do not get enough vitamins from the foods they eat and sunlight, it is important to take a vitamin D supplement to avoid a deficiency leading to osteoporosis.

Too Much Caffeine: If you are drinking more than two cups of coffee per day, there is a chance that you are leaching precious calcium from your bones. To be honest, it really doesn't matter if your caffeine comes from coffee, soda, energy drinks or some other source. Too much caffeine is detrimental to your long term bone health.

Long Term Steroid Use: The use of steroid medications to treat conditions such as seizure disorders, some cancers, gastric reflux and organ transplants have been linked to a higher incidence of osteoporosis.

Irritable Bowel Syndrome: Any type of irritable bowel syndrome or irritable bowel disease puts you at greater risk of osteoporosis. This is because the inflammatory state of the bowels will interfere with the absorption of valuable bone nutrients such as calcium and vitamin D.

Inflammatory Health Conditions: It has been shown that people with certain inflammatory health conditions are at a greater risk of developing osteoporosis. These conditions include celiac disease, lupus, kidney disease, liver disease, diabetes, cancer, and rheumatoid arthritis.

Certain Medications: The list of medications that can contribute to bone loss is actually quite long. It is important to discuss the medications that you take with your medical care provider and weigh the potential side effects against the potential benefits. If the medication that you take puts you at a greater risk of bone loss, make a point of requesting a bone density test annually. Some of the more popular medications that might cause bone loss include, but are not limited to:

- *Aluminum containing antacids*
- *Cortisone*
- *Depo-Provera*
- *Dilantin*
- *Femera*

- *Heparin*
- *Lexapro*
- *Lithium*
- *Methotrexate*
- *Nexium*
- *Phenobarbitol*
- *Prednisone*
- *Prevacid*
- *Prilosec*
- *Prozac*
- *Tamoxifen*
- *Zoloft*

Regardless of your age, if you feel that you have any of the potential risk factors for osteoporosis, you should not hesitate to contact your medical care provider for a proper screening. Osteoporosis is a condition where early detection and awareness can change the course and the progression of the disease.

Symptoms

They say that osteoporosis is a silent disease because most people are not aware that they have it until they suffer a painful or debilitating injury, as a result of the condition. This is why it is so important to take measures to protect your bone health long before osteoporosis is able to become a reality. It is equally important to recognize the early signs of osteoporosis, as well as the signs that the disease has progressed. Here are the signs and warning symptoms that you might be suffering from osteoporosis.

Loss of Height: We sometimes might make jokes about how we become shorter as we age. The truth behind this is actually no joking matter at all. As osteoporosis sets in the vertebra in the spine begin to compress and collapse, resulting in a loss of height.

Back Pain: In the early stages of osteoporosis it is common to suffer from back pain to collapsed vertebra or even an undiagnosed fracture.

Stooped Posture with Rounded Shoulders: When you see someone, typically an elderly person with a hunched over posture accompanied by rounded shoulders, this is a telltale sign of osteoporosis.

Bone Fractures: You might begin to experience bone fractures that don't seem to correspond to the incident that produced them. Seemingly small injuries can result in painful fractures and breaks. With severe bone mass loss, one might suffer a fracture from bumping into a piece of furniture, sneezing or even just the pressure from bending over.

Bone fracture of the Spine or Hip: These are two of the most common places for fractures in patients with osteoporosis. If you suffer from a fracture of one of these areas, it is worth looking at osteoporosis as the cause, especially if the incident leading to the fracture was relatively minor.

The Traditional Methods of Treating Osteoporosis

OSTEOPOROSIS

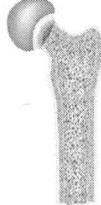
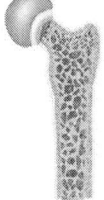

Normal Bone   Bone with Osteoporosis

When you and your doctor talk about the approaches for treating osteoporosis chances are that you will be provided a treatment plan that includes both pharmaceuticals and lifestyle adaptations. There are a variety of natural ways to treat osteoporosis; many of them are simple steps that you can take to prevent the development or advancement of the disease, especially in the earliest stages. The more natural approaches for treating osteoporosis include exercise, nutrition and supplementation.

Although surgery is sometimes required to repair damage caused by osteoporosis, surgery is not a treatment for the disease itself. There is a number of medications that are prescribed to prevent and treat osteoporosis, most of which work to slow the rate at which the bone tissue is reabsorbed. These medications are called antiabsorptives. In this section we will briefly describe each of them. If you have any questions about the medication that you are taking, become concerned about side effects or wonder if it is the best medication for you, please speak with your medical care provider immediately to discuss your concerns and possible alternatives.

Medications Used to Treat Osteoporosis

Bisphosphonates

Known by the brand names of Actonel, Boniva, Binosto, Fosamax and Reclast

This group of medications slows bone loss, increased bone density and helps prevent against bone fractures. This is accomplished by inhibiting the cells that are responsible for the degradation of bone material. Although each of these medications works very similarly, there are very strict instructions on how to take each of them. Some of them are once weekly medications, while other ones such as Boniva should only be taken once a month. Reclast is the one medication in this group that is administered through an IV once a year. Reclast is said to protect the most vulnerable areas of the body by reducing fractures to the spine, hips and wrists. If taken improperly, these medications can cause severe stomach upset, abdominal pain, heartburn and in more serious cases, ulcers of the esophagus.

Selective Estrogen Receptor Modifiers, also called SERMS

Known by the brand name Evista

At one point, estrogen replacement therapy was commonly prescribed as a method of treating osteoporosis in post menopausal women. Given that for many women the side effects of estrogen replacement therapy can be severe, it is rarely prescribed as a treatment for osteoporosis alone. A class of drugs called selective estrogen receptor modifiers act like estrogen in the body and help to maintain bone structure and prevent tissue loss. This class of drugs has been shown to not carry with it the same increased risks for breast and uterine cancer that come with estrogen replacement, and therefore is considered a safer alternative for post menopausal women. These medications are not recommended for premenopausal women. The most common side effects of these medications include hot flashes and the potential for blood clot formation.

Parathyroid Hormone
Known by the brand name of Forteo

A synthetic version of a natural occurring parathyroid hormone, this medication is a self administered daily injectable that can be taken for up to two years. Low doses of this medication can increase bone density and it is a preferred option for both men and postmenopausal women who are at an elevated risk for bone fractures because it is shown to not only promote the growth of new bone tissue but also increase bone mineral density. Typical side effects include nausea, dizziness and muscle cramps.

Biological Therapy
Known by the brand name of Prolia

Prolia is the first biological therapy to be approved for use as a treatment option for osteoporosis. It is a lab produced human monoclonal antibody. It works by shutting down the processes in the body that are responsible for the loss of bone tissue. At this point in time Prolia is not widely prescribed. It is indicated for postmenopausal women for whom other treatment methods have proved to be ineffective and are at an increased risk of bone fracture.

Calcitonin
Known by the brand name of Miacalcin

This medication is prescribed as an alternative for women who are unable to take estrogen related medications and those who are unable to tolerate or are unaffected by bisphosphonates. While not as effective as the bisphosphonates, it does work to slow the progression of bone loss and reduce bone fractures, especially those to the spinal area.

Hormone Replacement Therapy

Estrogen, either by itself or combined with progesterone, has been used to as an osteoporosis treatment to increase calcium absorption and reduce the potential for bone fractures. Estrogen replacement is seldom used with the sole purpose of treating osteoporosis because of the increased risk of certain breast and uterine cancers. The bone health properties are beneficial for menopausal women who are prescribed hormone replacement therapy indications other than osteoporosis. Some doctors prescribe a combination of estrogen and progesterone because it has been thought that the progesterone counters the carcinogenic effects of the estrogen. However, studies show that the combination of the two also increases the risk of certain cancer along with a higher risk of coronary disease and stroke. It is important to talk to your doctor about the potential side effects, your personal risk factors and then compare that against the perceived benefits before making a decision to begin hormone replacement therapy.

Natural Approaches to Osteoporosis Care

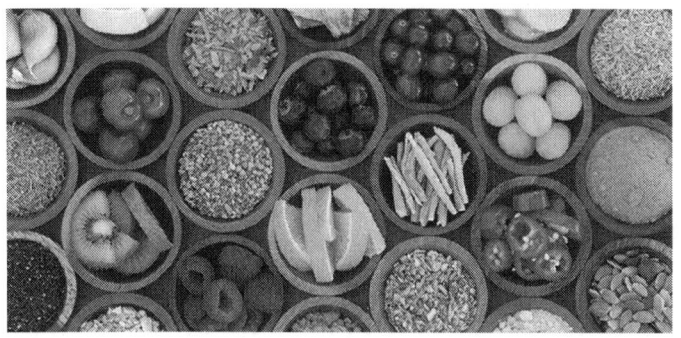

Whether or not you and your health care provider decide to use pharmaceuticals as one method of treating your osteoporosis, you are going to want to add complimentary natural treatments. These treatments will include lifestyle changes such as giving up bad habits, focusing on nutrition and exercise. We will discuss nutritional aspects, along with supplementation and exercise a little later in this book. Here, we would like to take a little time to talk about some of the other natural approaches to osteoporosis care.

Stress Reduction

When you are stressed your body produces a hormone called cortisol. During occasional periods of stress, the increase in cortisol is beneficial. However, when you are experiencing chronic stress over an extended period of time cortisol can have many effects that are detrimental to your health. Research shows that when cortisol levels are elevated over an extended period of time that bone health suffers. Of all of the factors that can contribute to the development of osteoporosis, stress related cortisol does not top the list. However, when you are vulnerable to developing osteoporosis, or already have the disease, the extra cortisol can accelerate the progression. Bone health aside, stress is bad for your body in so many ways. One of the best things that you can do for both your physical and mental health is to find ways to reduce the stress that comes into your life as well as discovering ways to deal with the stress that is simply unavoidable.

When we feel stressed it is also most often the case that we feel we have no more available energy to give. Yet, we continue to pile more onto our already full plates. The last person that you are likely to devote any of your time or energy to is yourself. This compounds to only make the stress worse and puts your health in a very vulnerable state. Additionally, when you are stressed you are more likely to be distracted and therefore more susceptible to accidents and clumsiness. If you are suffering from bone loss, this is a combination that you absolutely want to avoid.

The truth is that we all feel stress on some level from time to time, and many of us experience it daily. Some amount of stress is a necessary part of life. Stress can come from both negative and positive situations. Since stress itself is unavoidable, it becomes necessary to learn how to effectively cope with it, even if that means putting some of your other obligations aside and taking the time to focus on yourself and your health each day. There are multiple ways that you can learn to deal with stress more effectively. Because each one of us has different stress triggers and each one of us copes a little differently, the method that you choose will be highly individualized to you.

There is no one solution fits all when it comes to stress reduction; however there are some well respected natural techniques that have proven over time to be very effective. You might not always recognize the stress load that you are carrying, especially if you have been dealing with chronic stress for some time. This is one of the reasons that you should adopt at least one of the following techniques regardless of whether or not you feel you actually need it. Here are just a few ideas of ways to reduce your daily stress load.

• Give yourself some priority time. It can be as little as fifteen to twenty minutes, but spend at least some time each day doing something that you genuinely enjoy. This might be a cup a tea while enjoying a silent room or watching the morning birds outside your window. It might be a quick jog, steamy hot shower, doing a puzzle, playing a game, talking with a friend, etc. It can be easy to lose track of the small things in life that give you pleasure. When you take the time to introduce these things back into your life, even in small amounts, it helps to keep the rest of your life and the events taking place in proper perspective. I actually recommend taking some priority time at least twice a day, once in the morning and once in the evening, or whenever you need it. This gives you a little break to look forward to at least twice a day. If you think you just don't have the time or are too tired, think again. Even the busiest person can find a few minutes to go into a room, shut the door and just be by themselves if that is all that is available to you. There really isn't anything that you can accomplish in that same amount of time that is more important than your own health.

- Talk it out. When you internalize stress, it becomes magnified. Just the simple act of verbally sharing what you are experiencing can help to lighten the load. You might be most comfortable talking to a close friend or loved one, or you might prefer the advice and counsel of a non involved party, such as a therapist. Whatever works for you, seek it out and begin speaking. You might be surprised at some of the solutions that present themselves to you once you begin vocalizing. What should you do if you feel that you don't have anyone in your life that you can talk to or are dealing with something so personal or private that you just do not want to share it with another person? Share it with the universe. Find a quiet spot and simply start talking to the air, spirit or religious entity that you are connected to. Just vocalizing it helps to get some of the stress out of your body and give you a clearer perspective.

• Write it out. Journaling or blogging about the stressful events in your life is therapeutic in very much the same way as talking it out with another person. The added benefit of journaling is that you can look back on your writings and notice patterns, or which solutions worked and which ones didn't. Journaling provides opportunities for growth through retrospection.

• Join groups. People with active social lives and more social connections feel less stress. Interaction with other people is necessary for emotional health. Even if you are not a person that enjoys groups, chances are that even though you place high value on your solitude that you still appreciate and enjoy the company of honest friends. If you are going through a difficult time in your life, join a support group where you can interact with others going through the same thing. You might also look at joining groups with similar interests, such as a sport or crafting hobby, church group, reading group, etc. Even taking a class that interests you can give you the opportunity to meet people that you can connect with and take your mind off of the stressors in your life.

• Work it out. Physical exercise is a great way to reduce stress. As a bonus you will have more energy to deal with the stressors in your life, and weight bearing exercises are great for bone health. If all you have to give is fifteen minutes for stretches in the morning, then start there. Some exercise is better than none at all. There is a delicate balance between pushing yourself and respecting your limits when it comes to exercise. Begin by making it a priority to just get moving, and then build your strength and endurance from there. If you are dealing with osteoporosis, your exercise routine should be gentle and tailored to your specific needs in order to avoid unnecessary injury.

• Try the tried and true. You probably already know of many popular stress reduction techniques. The reason that you know about them is because they work. Stress reducers such as mediation, yoga, mindfulness, the use of essential oils, etc. are popular options because they are effective. If there is one or more of these techniques that you have been wanting to try, now is the time to do it.

Essential Oils

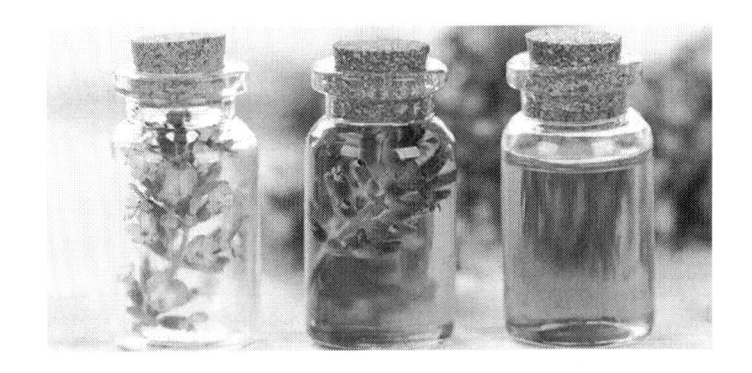

Since osteoporosis is a disease of bone degradation, you might not have expected that there are essential oils that help in the treatment of the disease. While it is true that you cannot magically reach into your body and apply essential oils to your fragile or broken bones, essential oils can offer many comforts when used topically.

Although scientific research is lacking, there is speculation that the topical application of some essential oils can actually stimulate bone tissue growth. Even with this, one of the most important applications of essential oils concerning osteoporosis is that they can provide soothing pain relief and help to reduce inflammation that can make the condition worse. The best essential oils to use for osteoporosis symptoms include:

• *Wintergreen*
• *Eucalyptus*
• *Cypress*
• *Frankincense*
• *Oregano*

Some of these oils, especially the ones with warming properties, can harm your skin when applied directly. You should always dilute your essential oils in some type of carrier oil before applying them to your skin. Carrier oils should be plant based. Examples of carrier oils include coconut oil, olive oil, almond oil, rice bran oil, avocado oil, and evening primrose oil, among others.

Ten to fifteen drops of essential oil to one ounce of carrier oil is usually enough to provide a therapeutic strength application. Start with the lowest amount of essential oils and add a few more drops if you like once you know how you tolerate the oils.

To use the oils, rub your dilution into the parts of your body that hurt, or are most susceptible to injury, such as your arms, wrist, hips and back. You can do this both morning and night. You can also add several drops of oil to a nice relaxing bath for an all over soothing treatment.

Herbs

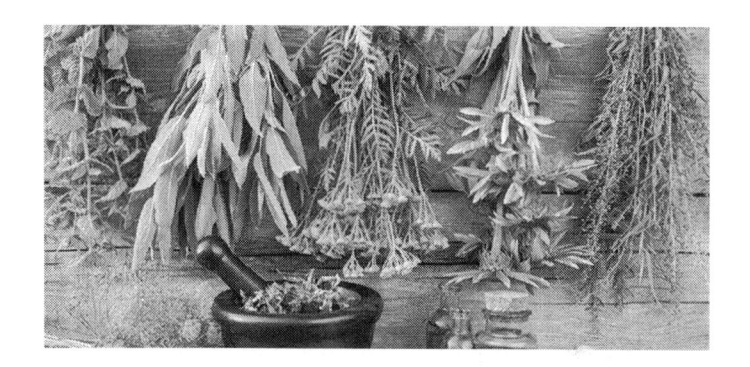

There are certain herbs that have favorable properties for treating osteoporosis. Many of the herbs that are beneficial for bone health provide estrogen like effects. Because herbs do not undergo the same type of scientific scrutiny that pharmaceuticals do, the long term effects of these estrogen like properties are not always known. Because herbs are readily available and do not carry with them the same research as other medications, they are often viewed as not being as potent as their pharmaceutical counterparts. The fact is that herbs can be just as potent as traditional medications, and that includes all of the benefits and the side effects. It is important to discuss the use of herbs with your medical care provider, especially if you are already taking medication for osteoporosis, are taking other medications, especially those that have a thinning effect on the blood, or have any type of estrogen sensitive condition or concern. The following herbs are among the best for addressing the effects of osteoporosis.

Black Cohosh: This herb is often used by women to relieve menopausal discomforts. Black cohosh contains estrogen like substances called phytoestrogens, which mimic the effect of estrogen in the prevention of bone loss. Because of the phytoestrogens, this herb might not be the best choice if you are at an elevated risk of or have experienced estrogen sensitive cancers.

Red Clover: Another herb with estrogen like properties, red clover contains isoflavones which work to slow and prevent bone loss. The same precautions that apply to black cohosh also apply to red clover.

Kelp: the dried extract of kelp is rich in minerals which can help build bone strength.

Oat Straw: Helps to stabilize and boost the hormone levels that are necessary for bone cell growth and repair.

Horsetail: This herb contains natural silicone which is thought to be beneficial for increasing bone strength.

Quitting Bad Health Habits

We have already mentioned in the previous sections that certain lifestyle habits can increase your risk for developing osteoporosis. If you are looking for an all natural approach to treating your osteoporosis, the first thing you should do is take a look at any poor lifestyle habits that you may have and develop a plan for changing them. The lifestyle factors that can have the biggest impact on your health include smoking, excessive alcohol consumption, excessive caffeine consumption, living a sedentary lifestyle and obesity.

Smoking, alcohol and caffeine can actually pull extra calcium from your bones. In addition to making you more vulnerable to osteoporosis, these habits can actually counteract the effects of the medication that you are taking, making them less effective. If you smoke, talk with your doctor about the best approach for reducing the amount you smoke and then eventually quitting. Alcohol and caffeine do not pose as much of a risk when consumed in moderate amounts. Limit yourself to no more than one or two of either of these drinks per day. One alcoholic drink is considered to be one ounce of hard liquor, one six ounce beer or one four ounce glass of wine, Caffeine should be limited to no more than the equivalent of two cups of coffee per day.

Your Diet and Osteoporosis: The Nutrition You Need to Build and Repair Bone Health

The number one way that you can prevent or treat osteoporosis is through dietary means. When you first speak to your doctor, you will come to a decision regarding medications. There is no question that sometimes medications are the best route, especially for people with more advanced, severe bone disease. In these cases, attention to a bone building diet will compliment your drug therapy. If your case is mild or you are just beginning to consider the long term health of your bones, then a more natural dietary approach can be the first line of defense against osteoporosis.

Eating to build and repair your bones really isn't very difficult at all. The focus is on incorporating whole, natural foods into your diet while eliminating processed foods which are bad for your body in general. You know that calcium is the number one component of a diet that builds bones. You have probably heard from childhood that a glass of milk builds strong bones. This is definitely true. Calcium is essential for bone formation. In addition to calcium your body also requires vitamin D, vitamin K and magnesium. Here, in this section we will address those specific bone friendly requirements and discuss which foods to add more of into your diet and which ones to avoid altogether.

Without question, the best way to get calcium is through the foods you eat. As a secondary line of caution, you may be advised to take a calcium supplement to compensate for any lack of calcium from your daily food choices. You need to be careful with calcium supplementation because too much of a good thing, in this case calcium, can cause more harm than good. Additionally, some research is addressing a connection between calcium supplementation and a possible increased risk of heart disease. This connection requires more research and there is no reason to put down your calcium supplement just yet. Rather, this possible connection does give us enough reason to favor calcium rich foods over supplements whenever possible.

Most people do not take in nearly enough calcium to prevent bone deterioration. In fact, it is estimated the majority of women take in only one third to one half of the calcium that their bodies need on a daily basis. When you do not take in enough calcium either through food sources or through supplementation, your body then pulls it from the only other resource it has; your bones. This is why adequate calcium intake on a daily basis is so important. Here are the recommended daily intake amounts of calcium. For reference, one eight-ounce glass of milk, either skim or whole, contains approximately 300 milligrams of calcium.

- **Children**   1,200 milligrams per day
- **Adults 19-50** 1,000 milligrams per day
- **Adults 50+**   1,200 milligrams per day

In order to reach these target amounts of calcium, the average adult should consume three to four servings of calcium rich foods per day. Some of the best dietary sources of calcium include:

Dairy Products: Low fat dairy products contain just as much calcium as the full fat varieties. So, unless you have specific dietary needs that call for the more fat rich options, choose low fat whenever possible. Examples of calcium rich dairy include milk, cheeses and yogurt.

Vegetables: Dark, leafy green vegetables are the highest in calcium. Examples include spinach, kale, collard greens, mustard greens, turnip greens and broccoli. Other vegetables such as potatoes, sweet potatoes, artichokes, red bell peppers, green bell peppers and Brussels sprouts contain complimentary nutrients such as vitamin C, vitamin K and magnesium.

Fruits: Some bone friendly fruits that either contain calcium or other nutrients that aid in the absorption of calcium include: figs, raisins, prunes, papaya, oranges, banana and pineapple.

Fish: Fish with small bones such as salmon or sardines, Fatty vitamin D containing fish such as salmon, mackerel, sardines and tuna.

Calcium fortified foods: examples include some juices, breakfast cereals and bread products.

Miscellaneous sources: almonds, blackstrap molasses, almonds, sesame seeds, tofu, black eyed peas.

Some people find it difficult to add in so many servings of calcium rich foods into their diets, especially if they are trying to avoid dairy products for dietary or sensitivity reasons. If you are lactose intolerant or dairy sensitive, make a point of including as many non dairy sources of calcium as possible into your diet and speak with your medical care provider about the best choice of supplementation for you. If you don't have any food sensitivities but are worried that you might not be able to add in enough calcium rich foods into your diet, try some of these tips for increasing your daily calcium intake:

• Fortify your meals and snacks such as soups and smoothies with a tablespoon of dry, powdered milk.

• When making soups and sauces, substitute at least part of the required liquid with milk or cream.

• Use milk instead of water when making hot cereals, cooking rice or making tea.

- Fortify your baked goods such as muffins and pancakes with milk or yogurt.

- Use nonfat, plain yogurt to add extra creaminess and texture to foods such as mashed potatoes, guacamole, savory dips, casseroles, etc.

- Try fancy, new cheeses as part of dessert or snack plate and pair them with figs.

- Change the proportions of your plate and take extra large servings of calcium rich foods.

- Make a calcium rich meal by topping fresh, dark leafy greens with salmon and your choice of bone healthy fruits and vegetables.

- Chop up calcium rich greens and add them to practically any dish, even smoothies.

- Prepare easy to grab calcium rich snacks ahead of time, such as a handful of almonds, paired with papaya and a nibble of your favorite cheese.

- Make homemade bone stock and add a little calcium to the broth as it is cooking to help pull more calcium from the bones used.

Calcium and complimentary nutrients are essential to a bone healthy diet. However, eating to protect your bones involves an equal amount of knowing what to avoid in your diet. Certain foods are not only bad for your overall health, but can actually cause bone loss and counteract the positive actions that you are taking against osteoporosis. The main foods to avoid include:

- *Sweetened Beverages: This is especially true for sodas that contain high amounts of phosphorus which can actually pull calcium from the bones. In addition, sugar causes inflammation which has been shown to accelerate osteoporosis.*

• *Processed Foods: Most processed foods are high in sodium, which is detrimental to bone health.*

• *Alcohol*

• *Caffeine*

Excessive amounts of acidic foods: examples include red meat, processed meats, foods made from white flour such pasta and bread, most high sodium foods.

Before you go and start making long, complicated grocery and meal lists that you are less likely to stick to long term, take a step back and really look at the above information. Do you notice something? The foods that you need to keep your body and your bones healthy are wholesome and all natural. Yes, there are certain foods that are higher in calcium and other nutrients that your bones needs and yes, you need to incorporate more of them into your diet. However, when you focus on clean, healthy eating, you will be surprised at how naturally and effortlessly you are able to fill your plates with healthy foods that you and your bones need. Keep this in mind as you prepare to eat to treat and prevent osteoporosis. Eat as naturally as possible, choose organic whenever your budget allows and enjoy the true natural flavors of nature's healing foods.

Easy Bone Building Recipes

Do you think that a bone friendly diet is about nothing more than drinking milk and snacking on cheese? Think again, because there are practically limitless options for delicious, calcium rich and bone friendly meals. Your creativity will determine your culinary limits. Here are just a few recipes to get you started.

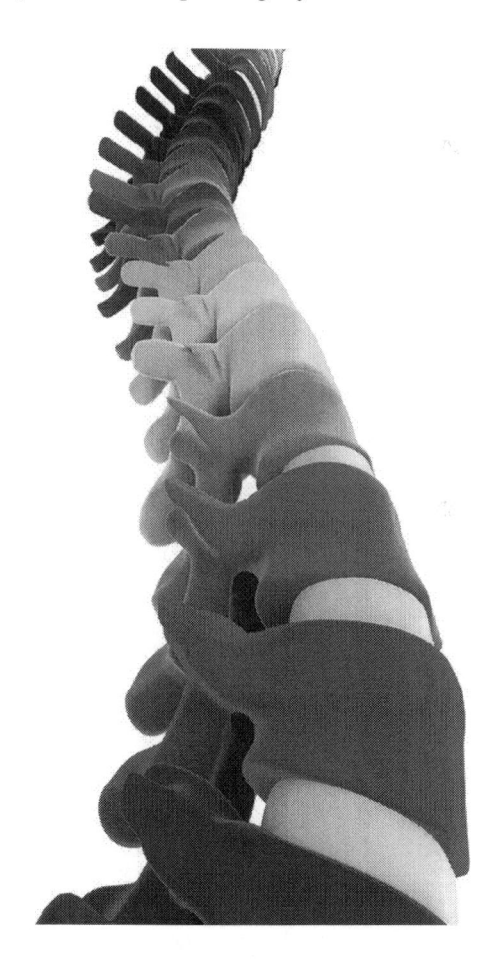

Decadent Chocolate Smoothie

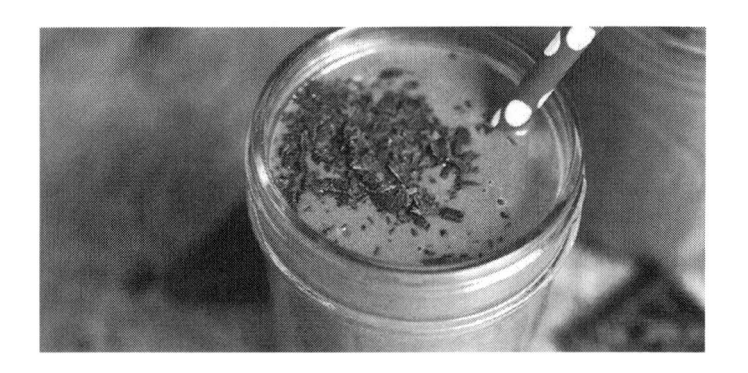

Servings: 2-3

Ingredients:

2 cups low fat vanilla yogurt

1 cup skim milk

1 teaspoon pure vanilla extract

½ teaspoon cinnamon

2 tablespoons dark cocoa powder

¼ cup dark chocolate chips

¼ cup almonds

1 cup ice

Additional shaved chocolate for garnish, optional

Directions:

Place all of the ingredients in a blender, or smoothie maker. Blend until smooth.

Transfer to well chilled glasses and serve immediately.

Blackberry Papaya Smoothie

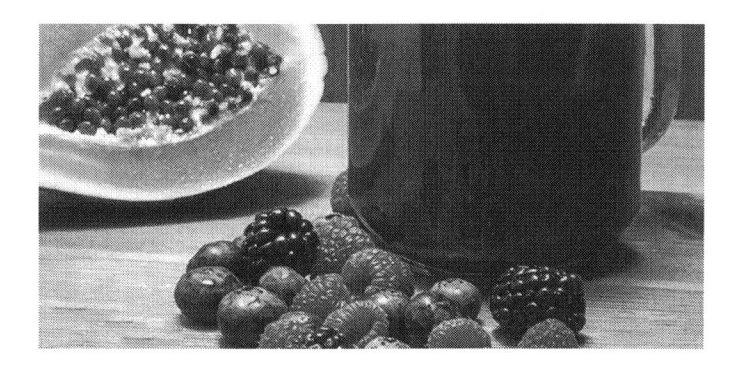

Servings: 2-3

Ingredients:

2 cups non fat vanilla yogurt

1 cup almond milk

1 cup papaya, cubed

1 cup blackberries

2 teaspoons fresh grated ginger

¼ cup fresh mint

1 tablespoon fresh lime juice

1 cup ice

Directions:

Place all of the ingredients in a blender of smoothie maker. Blend until smooth. Transfer to well chilled glasses and serve immediately.

Spinach Artichoke Portabellas

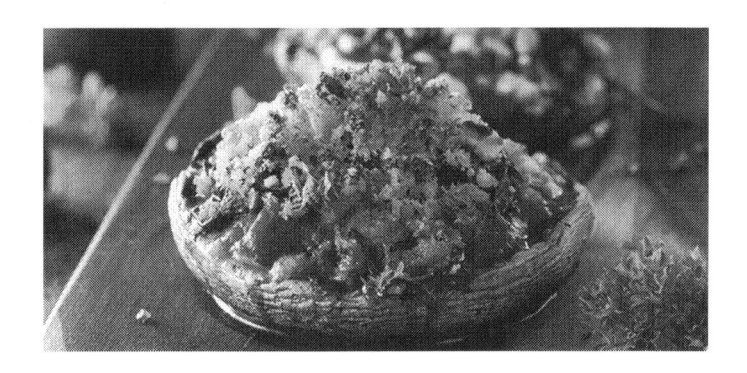

Servings: 4

Ingredients:

4 large portabella mushroom caps

1 tablespoon olive oil, divided

1 teaspoon coarse ground black pepper

4 cups fresh spinach, torn

1 cup artichoke hearts, chopped

½ cup red bell pepper, diced

2 cloves garlic, crushed and minced

1 cup skim ricotta cheese

½ cup provolone cheese, shredded

½ cup fresh grated parmesan cheese

1 teaspoon fresh oregano

1 teaspoon nutmeg

Directions:

Preheat the oven to 450°F and line a baking sheet with aluminum foil.

Brush both sides of the mushrooms with olive oil and place the mushroom caps on the baking sheet, gill side up.

Place the baking sheet in the oven and bake the mushrooms for approximately 20 minutes.

While the mushrooms are baking, add the remaining olive oil to a skillet over medium heat.

Add in the garlic and red bell pepper. Sauté for 2 minutes. Next, add in the spinach and artichokes and sauté for an additional 3-5 minutes.

Remove the skillet from the heat and stir in the ricotta cheese, provolone cheese, oregano and nutmeg. Set aside until the mushrooms come out of the oven.

Remove the mushrooms from the oven and allow them to cool enough to be handled. Spoon equal amounts of the spinach mixture into each mushroom cap.

Cover with a sprinkling of fresh grated parmesan.

Place the mushrooms back in the oven and bake until the tops are golden, approximately 10 minutes.

Ultimate Stuffed Cheese Quesadilla

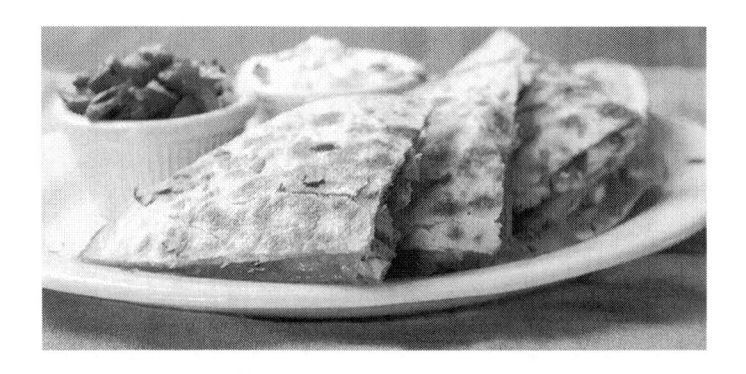

Servings: 2

Ingredients:

4 large whole grain flour tortillas

1 cup Mexican melting cheese, shredded

1 cup low fat pepper jack cheese, shredded

1 cup black beans, cooked

1 cup green bell pepper, sliced thin

1 cup mushrooms, sliced

1 poblano pepper, seeded and sliced

1 jalapeno pepper, seeded and sliced

½ cup avocado, cubed

¼ cup low fat plain yogurt

¼ cup fresh cilantro

Directions:

Spray a large skillet with cooking spray and heat over medium.

Add the green bell pepper, mushrooms, poblano pepper and jalapeno pepper to the skillet and sauté until crisp tender.

Add the black beans to the skillet and toss until warmed.

While the vegetables are sautéing, combine the avocado, plain yogurt and cilantro in a blender or food processor and blend until creamy.

Remove the sautéed vegetables from the skillet and set aside.

Lay one of the tortillas in the skillet and sprinkle with one half of the Mexican melting cheese. Top this with one half of the vegetable mixture, followed by half of the pepper jack cheese.

Spoon a desired portion of the avocado cream sauce over the top of the cheese and then top with another tortilla. Cook for 3-5 minutes per side until the cheese is melted.

Remove from the skillet and slice into wedges before serving.

Bone Building Salad

Servings: 4

Ingredients:

4 cups spinach, chopped

2 cups escarole

½ lb. pancetta, diced

1 cup blue cheese crumbles

1 cup dried figs, chopped

1 tablespoon shallots, diced

1 tablespoon fresh thyme

¼ cup champagne vinegar

2 tablespoons olive oil

1 tablespoon Dijon mustard

2 tablespoon pomegranate juice

1 tablespoon pure maple syrup

Directions:

Toss the spinach and escarole together and transfer to a large salad bowl or individual serving plates.

Place the pancetta in a skillet over medium heat. Sauté until the edges are browned and crisp. Remove the pancetta from the skillet and set aside to drain off any excess oil.

In a bowl combine the shallots, thyme, champagne vinegar, olive oil, Dijon mustard, pomegranate juice and maple syrup. Whisk together until well blended and slightly emulsified.

Decorate the salad greens with the crisp pancetta, chopped figs and bleu cheese crumbles.

Drizzle the desired amount of the dressing over the salad before serving.

Serve with additional dressing on the side, if desired.

Spicy Philly Enchiladas

Servings: 4

Ingredients:

8-12 flour tortillas, depending on size

2 cups cooked chicken, shredded

1 tablespoon olive oil

1 cup onion, sliced

1 cup green bell pepper, sliced

1 cup portabella mushrooms, sliced

3 cloves garlic, crushed and minced

1 cup tomatoes, diced

¼ cup canned green chilies

2 cup low fat milk

2 tablespoon flour

2 tablespoons butter

1 teaspoon cayenne powder

1 teaspoon smoked paprika

1 teaspoon onion powder

2 cups Swiss cheese

Directions:

Preheat the oven to 350° and lightly oil an 8x8 baking dish.

Add the olive oil to a skillet over medium heat. To the skillet add the onion and green bell pepper, and sauté for 2-3 minutes.

Next, add in the garlic, portabella mushrooms, tomatoes and canned green chilies. Continue sautéing for an additional 3-4 minutes.

Add in the chicken and toss until warmed.

In a separate saucepan, melt the butter over medium heat. Once the butter is melted, sprinkle in the flour and whisk until a paste forms.

Slowly, add in the milk and continue whisking until a sauce forms. Season the sauce with cayenne powder, smoked paprika and onion powder. Continue cooking, stirring frequently, until the sauce thickens.

Remove the sauce from the heat and spread about ¼ of it in the bottom of the baking dish.

Take each tortilla and fill it with an equal portion of the filling mixture. Roll the tortillas and place them face down in the baking dish. Pour the remaining sauce over the enchiladas and top with the Swiss cheese.

Place the baking dish in the oven and bake for 20-25 minutes, or until the cheese is melted and lightly browned.

Stuffed Endive

Servings: 4

Ingredients:

12 endive leaves, trimmed

½ cup low fat cream cheese

½ cup crème fraiche

1 tablespoon fresh chives

1 tablespoon capers

½ lb. salmon lox

1 lemon, sliced

1 tablespoon fresh thyme, chopped

Directions:

In a blender or food processor combine the cream cheese, crème fraiche, chives and capers. Blend until creamy.

Using a pastry bag, pipe equal amounts of the creamy mixture into each of the endive leaves.

Top each leaf with the salmon lox, a slice of fresh lemon and a sprinkling of fresh thyme before serving.

Spaghetti Squash Italiano

Serves: 4

Ingredients:

2 spaghetti squash

¼ cup seasoned bread crumbs

1 tablespoon olive oil

1 cup onion, diced

2 cups spinach, chopped

2 cloves garlic, crushed and minced

1 teaspoon oregano

¼ cup fresh basil

1 cup fresh mozzarella cheese

1 cup skim ricotta cheese

1 cup marinara sauce

Directions:

Preheat the oven to 425°F and line a baking sheet with aluminum foil.

Cut the spaghetti squash in half, brush with olive oil and place cut side down on the baking sheet. Place the squash in the oven and bake for 30-40 minutes, or until tender.

While the squash is baking add the olive oil to a skillet over medium heat. Add in the onion, spinach and garlic. Sauté for 3-5 minutes, or until tender.

Season the vegetables with oregano and basil, and then add in the marinara sauce. Reduce the heat to low and simmer for 10-15 minutes.

Remove the squash from the oven and let cool until they can be handled.

Lightly oil and 8x8 inch baking dish and reduce the heat of the oven to 350°F.

Scoop out the spaghetti squash insides and add them directly to the skillet with the sauce. Toss to coat.

Next, add in the ricotta cheese and mozzarella cheese and mix.

Transfer to the baking dish and top with seasoned bread crumbs.

Place the baking dish in the oven and bake for 20-25 minutes, or until bubbly and golden brown.

Supplements for Osteoporosis Care

There is no question that the best place to get your osteoporosis fighting nutrients is through the foods that you choose to nourish your body with. Sometimes though, that can be difficult or even impossible. If you are unable to reach your dietary needs through food along, then supplementation is your next best bet. Additionally, there are supplements that you can take to help prevent bone loss that you cannot get from food sources. Here is a comprehensive list of the best supplements to include in your osteoporosis care regimen.

Calcium: In the previous section we discussed how dietary calcium is superior to supplementary calcium. There is a wide variety of calcium rich foods to add to your diet, however, you simply might not be able to meet your dietary needs through diet along, or your doctor may advise additional supplementation based on your individual condition. When shopping for a calcium supplement it is important to know that there are several different types to choose from.

Calcium citrate: This is the preferred source of calcium because it is the most easily absorbed form and therefore more of it is readily available for your body to utilize. The only downside is that sometimes calcium citrate can be slightly costlier.

Calcium phosphate: The second best choice for supplementation, this form of calcium is easily absorbed and causes little stomach upset.

Calcium carbonate: This is the least expensive option, but not as easily absorbed and can sometimes cause gastrointestinal upset.

Calcium carbonate is the type of calcium that is added to chewable antacids such as Tums or Rolaids. This type of calcium supplementation is good if you are just trying to reinforce your already sufficient calcium intake. However, for full supplementation, another form should be chosen.

When taking calcium supplements, note that your body can only absorb so much at any one time. For this reason, it is wise to break up your calcium supplementation over at least two doses and do not take with foods that already contain calcium, as your body may not benefit from the total amount of calcium in that situation. Take up to 1,000 milligrams of calcium daily.

Vitamin D: The second most important nutrient for osteoporosis care is vitamin D. Your body needs vitamin D in order to effectively utilize calcium. It also helps to promote bone mineralization. Most people are at least slightly deficient in vitamin D, otherwise known as the sunshine vitamin. The body is capable of producing vitamin D on its own when exposed to the ultra violet rays of sunshine. Vitamin D is also available from foods that have been fortified with the vitamin such as milk and breakfast cereals. Between a lack of exposure to the sun and the use of sunscreens, many people are not able to produce enough vitamin D naturally. The amount of sunlight exposure that you need to produce adequate vitamin D varies from person to person depending upon the natural coloring of their skin, their geographical location and environmental factors that might affect UV saturation. For this reason, it is advisable to take in vitamin D is supplement form. Vitamin D3 is the recommended form for supplementation. You may take anywhere from 800-4,000 IU of vitamin D daily, depending on your individual condition.

Speak with your health care provider before taking more than two 800 IU doses of vitamin D daily.

Vitamin K: This vitamin is essential for bone mineralization, by activating proteins that are responsible for building bone mass. You may already be getting enough vitamin K from your food sources, so check with your health care provider about whether or not vitamin K supplementation is right for you. You can take up to 100 mcg daily of vitamin K2.

Magnesium: This nutrient is necessary to help metabolize calcium to the fullest extent. You can take up to 500 mg of magnesium daily.

Omega 3 Fatty Acids: Also found in fish oil supplements, omega 3 fatty acids have been shown to improve calcium absorption, reduce the amount of calcium lost and improve bone strength and mass. You can take up to 4 grams per day.

Ipriflavone: This is a synthetic isoflavone that is derived from natural sources. Isoflavones can mimic the effect of estrogen in the body and therefore take estrogen's place when it begins to decline in menopausal women. You can take up to 600 milligrams of ipriflavone per day, but you should also speak to your doctor before you begin supplementation.

Keeping Physically Active to Keep Bones Strong

If you have osteoporosis, or any degree of weak bones, you might think that the last thing you need to be doing is any type of exercise, especially if you have been warned that even the slightest injury can turn into a major health problem. The truth is that yes, you do need to be extra cautious and take care to not injure yourself during physical activity, however, regular strength building exercises rate right up there with proper nutrition when it comes to ways of protecting and strengthening your bone health.

Research confirms that weight bearing exercises, the ones that actually put mild stress on your bones, help to prevent osteoporosis and make your bones stronger. This goes against common thought that you should avoid any type of stress on your bones. Examples of weight bearing exercises include gentle weightlifting, resistance training, squats, stair climbing, carrying groceries home from a walk to the store, yoga, walking, and some forms of dance, such as ballet. While it is best to begin exercising when you are younger, in order to build the strongest bones possible, it is never too late to begin an exercise routine, as long as it is tailored to your needs and osteoporosis health concerns.

Before you begin any exercise program, you should undergo a thorough examination by your medical care doctor. You will need to be evaluated on your general fitness, balance, muscular strength, range of motion and fracture risk. Your doctor may first advise a balance control program, especially if you have a high fracture risk. This will help you to securely maintain your balance throughout your exercise routine, which is very important in injury prevention.

There are a couple of different schools of thought regarding exercise for the osteoporosis patient. One thought is that you get your exercise in short bursts of no more than ten minutes, once or twice a day, or more if you can tolerate it. The other theory is that you need a solid twenty to thirty minutes of appropriate exercise on most days to build bone strength. My personal take on this is that you should talk to your doctor and make your decision based on what is best for your body at this present time.

A well rounded, osteoporosis fighting exercise routine is going to contain several different components. These components include weight bearing exercises, muscles strengthening exercises and non impact exercises. Here are some of the best exercises in each of those categories:

Weight Bearing Exercises: These types of exercises require you to work against gravity:

- *Outdoor terrain walking*
- *Treadmill walking*
- *Elliptical machines*
- *Stair climbing machines*
- *Low impact aerobics*

Muscle Building Exercises: Increased muscle strength reduces the risk of fractures and helps promote bone mineralization:

- *Free weights*
- *Weight machines*
- *Resistance bands*

Non Impact Exercises: These exercises help to maintain a higher level of fitness and help to develop the balance and coordination that are needed to avoid falls and injuries.

- *Yoga*
- *Pilates*
- *Stretching*

If you already have osteoporosis, it is important that you not put so much stress on your bones while exercising that you increase your chance of injury. If you have osteoporosis of the spine, do not lift more than twenty pounds until your bones are strengthened and your doctor advises it. Additionally, here are a few more tips that you can use to help protect yourself from injury while exercising to make your bones stronger.

- Start in a chair. Lift weights while sitting, straight backed, in a chair. This eliminates the need to bend at the waist from a standing position in order to lift or put down the weights.

- Start with an amount of weight that you feel comfortable with. Yes, the point is to build strength and in order to do that you are going to need to go outside your comfort level, but it is important to start gently in order to properly assess your physical strength. It can be easy to become overzealous at the beginning of a new exercise regimen. This will only result in unnecessary pain and possible injury.

- If outdoor terrain is too unstable for you and you do not have access to a treadmill, try marching in place. Make sure to keep your back straight and your abdominal muscles tight.

- Don't neglect any muscle groups. You may decide to work each muscle group every day, or you may devote one day to certain muscle groups and cover the others the next day. Whichever way you choose, make sure that you are equally strengthening all of your body.

If one muscle group becomes stronger than other, that part will automatically work harder, reducing the amount of work the weaker part of your body does. If you have ever walked with a different gate because of an injury and ended up sore, you can understand how favoring one part of your body can have negative consequences.

• Along the same line of not neglecting any muscle groups, make sure to strengthen your body symmetrically. What you do with one side of your body, you must do with the other.

• Use resistance band to help you maintain your balance when needed. You can also do exercises against a wall or with the support of solid, stable furniture if you are at an increased risk of fall or injury.

If it has been some time since you have exercised, or if you have never committed to a regular routine before, you should know that the hardest part is just getting started. Once you have spent one to two weeks with your new exercise routine, not only will your bones be growing stronger, but you will without a doubt notice the other beneficial aspects of regular exercise including increased energy, balanced appetite, improved mood and the ability to focus and concentrate more clearly. Regular exercise is a vital part of a healthy lifestyle and it is never too late to start, especially if you want to build and protect your bone health.

Conclusion

Osteoporosis is a disease that does not get the attention that it deserves. We often figure that it is an unavoidable aspect of aging and with that, do little about preserving our bone health while we still can. To be fair, this isn't all your fault. The seriousness of osteoporosis is overlooked by popular health resources with the claim that as long as you get your calcium you shouldn't be concerned. The fact is that you should be very concerned about osteoporosis because it can severely impact the quality of your life if left untreated. This book has been written to help you address your bone health needs, and to help you do so as naturally as possible. Diet, exercise and other natural remedies can be just as effective as pharmaceutical medications for some people. And for those people that absolutely need medications, the steps to bone health that are outlined in this book will only serve to reinforce and accelerate the results of the medication.

As always, you should speak with your doctor regarding any changes that you wish to make in the care of your osteoporosis, and that includes natural and gentle methods like the ones outlined in this book. Make sure that you have a medical care provider that is like minded and willing to work with you and your medical values when it comes to treating osteoporosis. It is never too late to get started, and what you do today can benefit you tomorrow. The only mistake is to sit and do nothing. I hope that this book helps you on the path to healing and stronger bone health.

Made in the USA
Middletown, DE
13 May 2021